Handbook of
Clinical Depression

Handbook of Clinical Depression

Editor
Nikhil Gurjar MBBS MD (Psychiatry)
Consulting Psychiatrist
Dr DY Patil Medical College
Navi Mumbai, Maharashtra, India
Email: nikhilgurjar92@gmail.com

Associate Editor
Nikhil Gautam MBBS MD (Psychiatry)
Assistant Professor
Department of Psychiatry
Christian Medical College Hospital
Ludhiana, Punjab, India
Email: nikhilgautamx@gmail.com

Contributing Author
Jatin Anand MBBS MD (Psychiatry)
Consulting Psychiatrist
Central Jail Hospital, Tihar
New Delhi, India

Foreword
DM Mathur

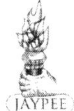

JAYPEE BROTHERS MEDICAL PUBLISHERS
The Health Sciences Publisher
New Delhi | London

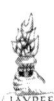

Jaypee Brothers Medical Publishers (P) Ltd

Headquarters
Jaypee Brothers Medical Publishers (P) Ltd
EMCA House, 23/23-B, Ansari Road, Daryaganj
New Delhi 110 002, India
Landline: +91-11-23272143, +91-11-23272703
+91-11-23282021, +91-11-23245672
Email: jaypee@jaypeebrothers.com

Corporate Office
Jaypee Brothers Medical Publishers (P) Ltd
4838/24, Ansari Road, Daryaganj
New Delhi 110 002, India
Phone: +91-11-43574357
Fax: +91-11-43574314
Email: jaypee@jaypeebrothers.com

Overseas Office
JP Medical Ltd
83 Victoria Street, London
SW1H 0HW (UK)
Phone: +44 20 3170 8910
Fax: +44 (0)20 3008 6180
Email: info@jpmedpub.com

Website: www.jaypeebrothers.com
Website: www.jaypeedigital.com

© 2023, Jaypee Brothers Medical Publishers

The views and opinions expressed in this book are solely those of the original contributor(s)/author(s) and do not necessarily represent those of editor(s) or publisher of the book.

All rights reserved. No part of this publication may be reproduced, stored or transmitted in any form or by any means, electronic, mechanical, photocopying, recording or otherwise, without the prior permission in writing of the publishers.

All brand names and product names used in this book are trade names, service marks, trademarks or registered trademarks of their respective owners. The publisher is not associated with any product or vendor mentioned in this book.

Medical knowledge and practice change constantly. This book is designed to provide accurate, authoritative information about the subject matter in question. However, readers are advised to check the most current information available on procedures included and check information from the manufacturer of each product to be administered, to verify the recommended dose, formula, method and duration of administration, adverse effects and contraindications. It is the responsibility of the practitioner to take all appropriate safety precautions. Neither the publisher nor the author(s)/editor(s) assume any liability for any injury and/or damage to persons or property arising from or related to use of material in this book.

This book is sold on the understanding that the publisher is not engaged in providing professional medical services. If such advice or services are required, the services of a competent medical professional should be sought.

Every effort has been made where necessary to contact holders of copyright to obtain permission to reproduce copyright material. If any have been inadvertently overlooked, the publisher will be pleased to make the necessary arrangements at the first opportunity.

Inquiries for bulk sales may be solicited at: jaypee@jaypeebrothers.com

Handbook of Clinical Depression

First Edition: **2023**

Reprint 2024

ISBN: 978-93-5696-152-4

Printed at Replika Press Pvt. Ltd.

Foreword

Depression is proving to be the major health problem of the current century. Although Depression has been there since the origin of mankind and likely to stay for the longest time, recently more and more number of individuals are facing it as an important health issue and approaching the mental health professionals for the solution.

With paucity of the professionals to treat depression like Psychiatrists and Clinical Psychologists, it is necessary for general practitioners to be aware of the presentation and approach toward depression. Since they are the initial point of clinical contact for a patient, the General Practitioners can identify the problem in an individual and be the first person to bring relief to the sufferer.

International reports suggest that almost one out of four patients attending any hospital or dispensary anywhere either have independent major depressive disorder or have associated symptoms reflecting comorbid depression, requiring management, to bring total improvement in the patient and their quality of life.

A General Practitioners, usually, because of insufficient and long past training in psychiatry or lack of availability of continued education in psychiatry courses would like to revise his/her knowledge of the problem and the recent advances in the management.

The authors of this book did justification by providing the necessary information about the epidemiology, phenomenology and modes of readily available and applicable methods to treat depression. The authors have also warned about the risk of suicide, which is not uncommon in the sufferers of depression and how to manage it at the right time.

The authors have avoided the jargon of unnecessary scientific terms and passed their message in simpler words to make it palatable.

I hope that this book would prove to be a positive asset to the reader and reward the authors with great satisfaction.

DM Mathur
Senior Consultant Psychiatrist
Eternal Hospital Jaipur
Former Professor and Head
Department of Psychiatry
Geetanjali Medical College and RNT Medical College
Udaipur, Rajasthan, India

Preface

High prevalence of illness, poor understanding of the illness, lack of adequate mental healthcare support and stigma, cause a lot of patients with depression to suffer unnecessarily. After COVID-19 a big surge in emergence of mental illnesses, particularly depression and anxiety were reported by various psychiatrists and mental health institutions. This led to increased awareness about the condition and further led to a decrease in hesitancy to seek treatment for the same. However, the ratio of mental health professionals required to meet the needs of the populations is highly skewed. There is a severe lack of mental health professionals like psychiatrists, clinical psychologists and psychiatric social workers.

Many persons with mental health issues find it more acceptable to speak about their problems with physicians and other clinicians, as there is still a stigma in seeking the help of psychiatrists directly. Therefore, it is important for physicians, general practitioners and clinicians of all specialties to have a working understanding of depression. This will help in identifying patients with depression correctly and providing them adequate guidance on how to go about the treatment of their problems. It will help facilitate treatment faster, decrease unnecessary suffering and can result in better outcomes for the patients and their families. This book will provide basic information about the illness characteristics, etiology and management which will help all clinicians understand the condition better and help in assessment, guidance and further management of patients.

Nikhil Gurjar

Acknowledgments

I am deeply indebted to my teachers in the field of psychiatry Professor Dr DM Mathur, Professor Dr Jitendra Jeenger, and Professor Dr Manu Sharma whose teachings have guided and inspired us to write this book. They have been instrumental in instilling in us a sense of why it is extremely important for us to educate all the persons whom we encounter who may be struggling with mental health problems since the nascent stages of our training in the world of psychiatry. It is because of these teachings that we feel duty bound to educate all the persons in our care along with their families about the nature of their illness, causes and implications.

I am also extremely grateful for all the help given to me by Professor Dr Kiran Godse. His mentorship, guidance, patient listening, and extremely practical and effective solutions have helped immensely while writing this book and this book would not have been possible without him.

I would like to thank my senior colleague Dr Chetan Vispute for his guidance. I would also like to thank my parents and my wife for their continuous support throughout this endeavor.

And last but not the least, I would like to thank my patients who constantly teach me and enhance my learning. I dedicate this book to all of them.

CHAPTER 1

Introduction

Nikhil Gautam

Depression is a common illness worldwide, with an estimated 3.8% of the population affected, which includes 5.0% adults and 5.7% adults older than 60 years. In India, the prevalence of depressive disorders in adults is around 3.3%. Approximately, 280 million people in the world are noted to have depression. In 2017, 45.7 million people had depressive disorders in India. Among the mental disorders that manifest predominantly during adulthood, the highest disease burden in India was caused by depressive and anxiety disorders with the highest contribution to disability adjusted life years due to mental disorders in India in 2017 was from depressive disorders (33.8%). Furthermore, depressive disorder has been ranked as the third cause of the burden of disease worldwide in 2008 by the World Health Organization (WHO), which has projected that this disease will rank first by 2030.

Depression is different from usual mood fluctuations of day-to-day life and short-lived emotional responses to challenges in life. Especially, when it is recurrent and has reached a moderate or severe intensity, depression can become a serious health condition. It may cause the affected person to suffer greatly and function poorly at work, at school and in the family.

At its worst, depression can lead to suicide. Over 700, 000 people die by suicide every year. Suicide is the fourth leading cause of death amongst 15–29-year-old. About two-thirds of all depressed patients contemplate about suicide, and 10–15% attempt suicide. Those that have been recently hospitalized with a suicide attempt or suicidal ideation have a higher lifetime risk of successful suicide than those never hospitalized for suicidal ideation.

Furthermore, there is a shortage of mental health personnel in India with two mental health workers and 0.3 psychiatrists per 100, 000 population, which is much lower than the global average. Additionally, the discriminatory attitude of the general population and healthcare workers toward people with mental illness and demand-side barriers such as the low perceived need for care, paucity of knowledge about mental disorders, and stigma attached to mental disorders are challenges that have yet to be addressed. Thus, task-sharing with non-specialists and appropriate training of general health practitioners and workers is the need of the hour to improve the mental health service provision. It is hoped that the information in this book can support this cause and help people better understand depression as a disorder and its management.

Depression is, by definition, a mood disorder, and disturbances of mood are at the core. Patients feel "bad" and may use words such as "sad," "blue," "not good," and "down," or similar words to describe this feeling. The term *depressed mood* or *dysphoria* is used to encompass

> **BOX 1:** Salient features of depression.
>
> - Sadness of mood, loss of pleasure in activities, which one enjoyed earlier, generalized lack of interest, easy fatiguability, and anxiety is often associated
> - Lack of energy, decreased concentration and efficiency
> - Lack of sleep, appetite and libido
> - Ideas of insufficiency, inadequacy and worthlessness, unexplained ideas of guilt, death wishes, suicidal ideas, and history of suicidal attempt
> - Symptoms should be present for a minimum duration of two weeks for a diagnosis to be made

these various depressive feelings. Some patients deny this depressed mood altogether, but instead, describe feeling unable to enjoy things that are usually enjoyable to them. We call this by the term *anhedonia* or a lack of pleasure. In addition to symptoms of dysphoria and anhedonia, many depressed patients might also report feeling anxious.

Patients having depression often present to the general practitioners and the physicians. These patients sometimes present with vague somatic symptoms or aches and pains in general clinical practice, for which no physical cause is found on assessment. During a depressive episode, a person experiences significant difficulty in personal, family, social, educational, occupational, and/or other important areas of functioning. A careful screening for depressive symptoms (as outlined under salient features) can elicit the diagnosis for depressive disorder **(Box 1)**.

■ SUGGESTED READING

1. India State-Level Disease Burden Initiative Mental Disorders Collaborators. The burden of mental disorders

across the states of India: the Global Burden of Disease Study 1990-2017. Lancet Psychiatry. 2020;7(2):148-61.
2. Kessler RC, Aguilar-Gaxiola S, Alonso J, Chatterji S, Lee S, Ustün TB. The WHO World Mental Health (WMH) Surveys. Psychiatrie (Stuttg). 2009;6(1):5-9.
3. Malhi GS, Mann JJ. Depression. Lancet. 2018;392(10161): 2299-2312.

CHAPTER 2

Etiology of Depression

Nikhil Gautam

INTRODUCTION

The etiology of depression is considered to be multifactorial and is not completely understood. It is not known exactly what causes depression, however, what is understood is that it results from a complex interaction of social, psychological, and biological factors. The purpose of this chapter is to review what is known or suspected about the causes of depression. Depressive symptoms such as sad mood, pessimism, and lethargy, are considered normal reactions to the struggles of everyday life. However, for some individuals, the intensity and persistence of depressive symptoms are not typical and can lead to illness. This chapter discusses some of the characteristics of individuals that may make them vulnerable, as well as the features of environments that are likely to provoke depression. The chapter also emphasizes the interplay between persons and environments—the ways in which, for example, stressful life events may provoke depression.

GENETIC FACTORS

Mood Disorders tend to run in families, and this has been proven by twin Studies. The twin studies data provide compelling evidence that genes explain only 50–70% of the etiology of mood disorders. The environment or other nonheritable factors must explain the remainder. Family data indicates that if one parent has a mood disorder, a child will have a risk of between 10 and 25 percent for mood disorder. If both parents are affected, then this risk roughly doubles. It is to be noted that it is the susceptibility to disease that is actually inherited and the not the disease itself. Gene-mapping studies of unipolar depression have also found very strong evidence of linkage to the locus for cyclic AMP response element-binding protein (CREB1) on chromosome 2.

BIOLOGICAL FACTORS

Biogenic Amines

There are three major amines that have played a role in causation of depression. The lack of monoamines namely serotonin, dopamine and noradrenaline availability at receptor sites in the brain can lead to depression. The fact that certain drugs and diseases that deplete monoamines (e.g., reserpine and Parkinson disease) cause depressive symptoms and antidepressants that cure said symptoms act on the monoamines (particularly catecholamines as noted above) led to the theory that depression is the result of deficiency or dysregulation in brain monoamines. Patients with suicidal impulses have shown low cerebrospinal fluid (CSF) concentrations of serotonin metabolites. Although this theory has become prevalent, several lines of evidence suggested it as an inadequate explanation for the etiology of depression.

Most notably, antidepressants take weeks to work, even though their presumed action of increasing monoamine levels happens quickly, often within hours after administration.

A number of studies have investigated the role of genetics in the serotonin-related genes in the etiology of depression. Research in individuals with changes in alleles of serotonin transporter (5-HTTLPR) gene experienced more depressive symptoms and higher rates of depressive disorder in response to stressful life events.

Neuroendocrine Regulation

Recent studies in depressed humans indicate that a history of early trauma is associated with increased hypothalamic pituitary adrenal (HPA) axis activity accompanied by structural changes (i.e., atrophy or decreased volume) in the cerebral cortex. Elevated HPA activity is a hallmark of the mammalian stress response and shows the role of chronic stress in biology of depression. There is also a correlation between the hypersecretion of cortisol and depression. Hypercortisolemia in depression suggests one or more of the following central disturbances: decreased inhibitory serotonin tone; increased drive from norepinephrine, acetylcholine, or corticotropin-releasing hormone; or decreased feedback inhibition from the hippocampus. Hypothyroidism is one of the most common disorders found in depression and should always be checked for. Approximately, 5–10% of patients evaluated for depression have previously undetected thyroid dysfunction, which is reflected by an elevated basal thyroid-stimulating hormone (TSH) level. Such abnormalities are often associated with elevated anti-thyroid antibody levels and, unless corrected with hormone replacement therapy, can lead to poor response to anti-depressive treatment.

Immune System Processes

Depressive disorders are associated with immunological abnormalities such as decreased lymphocyte proliferation in response to mitogens and other forms of impaired cellular immunity. There appears to be a link with clinical severity, hypercortisolism, and immune dysfunction. A possibility exists that chronic stressors might prime the immune system to make a heightened response to stress. Alternatively, chronic stress may interfere with the capacity of the immune system to return to baseline even after termination of a stressor, perhaps due to dysregulation of the HPA response and the production of glucocorticoids in response to stress. The inflammatory response may also contribute to symptoms of depression like disruptions in appetite, sleep, and social activity.

■ PSYCHOSOCIAL FACTORS

Adverse life events can trigger depression and often precede the development of symptoms. Life events that lead to feelings of entrapment and humiliation may be particularly relevant. One theory proposed to explain this observation is that the exposure to stress initially results in long-lasting changes in the brain's biology. These long-lasting changes may alter the functioning of various neurotransmitter and intraneuronal systems, changes that may include the loss of neurons and an excessive reduction in synapses. As a result, a person has a high risk of undergoing depression, even without an external stressor. The environmental stressor that is most often associated with the onset of depression is the loss of a spouse. Another risk factor is unemployment; persons out of work are three times more likely to report symptoms of an episode of major depression than those who are employed. Guilt may also play a role.

■ PSYCHOLOGICAL FACTORS

Cognitive Theory of Depression

According to cognitive theory people with depression tend to form have characteristic ways of interpreting events and circumstances that are excessively pessimistic, with perceptions of helplessness and hopelessness about changing or improving their situations. This way of thinking includes developing negative views about self, environment and future i.e., a cognitive triad of depression that consists of (1) views about the self —a negative perception of oneself, (2) about the environment—a tendency to experience the world as hostile and demanding, and (3) about the future—the expectation of failure and suffering.

Learned Helplessness

The learned helplessness theory of depression connects depressive phenomena to the experience of uncontrollable events in life. For example, when dogs in a laboratory were exposed to electrical shocks in a cage from which they could not escape, they showed behaviors that differentiated them from dogs that had not been exposed to such uncontrollable events. The dogs that were exposed to the shocks when placed in a new environment without the cage would not escape to stop the flow of electric shock even when put in a new situation without the cage. They remained passive and did not move. According to the learned helplessness theory, the shocked dogs learned that outcomes were independent of responses, so they had both decreased motivation (i.e., they would not attempt to escape the shock) and decreased emotional response (indicating decreased reactivity to the shock). This theory, as applied to human depression, notes that this phenomenon of helplessness in a depressed individual is thought to produce a loss of self-esteem after adverse external events.

ENDO-REACTIVE

Depression is diagnosed, respectively, when sadness is overly intense and continues beyond the expected impact of a stressful life event. Depressive disorders are conceptualized as endo-reactive i.e., once released due to external factors, they tend to persist autonomously in response to these factors. The term reactive depression which is known as adjustment disorder in current classification terminology signifies that the symptoms can be reversed with the removal from stressful situation which might be the cause.

SUGGESTED READING

1. Beck AT, Alford BA. Depression: Causes and treatment. University of Pennsylvania Press; 2009 Mar 25.
2. Boku S, Nakagawa S, Toda H, Hishimoto A. Neural basis of major depressive disorder: beyond monoamine hypothesis. Psychiatry Clin Neurosci. 2018;72(1):3-12.

3. Caspi A, Sugden K, Moffitt TE, Taylor A, Craig IW, Harington H, et al. Influence of life stress on depression: moderation by a polymorphism in the 5-HTT gene. Science. 2003; 301:386-9.
4. Flint J, Kendler KS. The genetics of major depression. Neuron. 2014;81(3):484-503.
5. Kendler KS, Kuhn JW, Vittum J, Prescott CA, Riley, B. The interaction of stressful life events and a serotonin transporter polymorphism in the prediction of episodes of major depression: a replication. Arch Gen Psychiatry.2005;62:529-35.
6. Kendler KS, Thornton LM, Gardner CO. Genetic risk, number of previous depressive episodes, and stressful life events in predicting onset of major depression. Am J Psychiatry. 2001;158:582-6.
7. Miller GE, Blackwell E. Turning up the heat: inflammation as a mechanism linking chronic stress, depression, and heart disease. Curr Dir Psychol Sci. 2006;15:269-72.
8. Sullivan PF, Neale MC, Kendler KS. Genetic epidemiology of major depression: review and meta-analysis. Am J Psychiatry. 2000;157(10):1552-62.
9. Tennant C. Life events, stress and depression: A review of the findings. Aust N ZJPsychiatry. 2002;36:173-82.

CHAPTER 3

Clinical Features of Depression

Nikhil Gurjar

■ INTRODUCTION

Depression or Major Depressive Disorder is characterized by a pervasive lowering of mood. The American Psychological Association defines mood as a disposition to respond emotionally in a particular way that may last for hours, days, or even weeks, perhaps at a low level and without the person knowing what prompted the state.

Simply put, the mood could be understood by asking a patient how he feels internally. A pervasive change in its quality, i.e., feeling sad most of the time is an indicator of pervasive mood change. A person's mood could be low because of many reasons which does not essentially indicate a morbid change, as it could be in response to a stressful life situation, grief or other similar factors.

A pathological mood change, however, could be distinguished from a normal mood state by the following factors:

- The response is *not proportionate* (or could be exaggerated) to an associated stressful situation or life event.

Clinical Features of Depression | 13

- When the person is *unable to feel reassured despite adequate support* about it.
- When the change in mood is *sustained for a long period of time*.
- If the persons mood change leads to *impaired judgement and decision making*.
- To understand this better, let us look at the example. Mr X has not been feeling good for a few days. When he goes to his office, he does not feel like working much. When his colleagues ask him why he seems so down these days, he tells them that this boss reprimanded him a few weeks ago for not meeting a deadline for his project. His friends proceed to tell him that it happens with everyone and that he should not take it too seriously. However, Mr X still appears to be sad most of the time. When his boss learns about this, he calls Mr X in his office and tells him that the project is over and that he should not continue to ponder on the events that transpired in the past and that he is doing a good job otherwise. But Mr X still does not feel better after talking to his boss. After a few weeks, he stops going to work. His family members, concerned by his behavior also try to motivate and encourage him, but Mr X just keeps saying that he feels he is not good enough to work at the office anymore. Mr X does not even try to apply for other jobs in spite of being unemployed for several months now.

This example helps us understand what a pathological mood state looks like.

Depressed mood is the hallmark feature of a Major Depressive Episode. It is also sometimes referred to as a sad, anguished, mournful, irritable or anxious feeling.

Some patients who are suffering from a milder severity of depression may deny this depressed mood and instead focus on physical symptoms such as headache, body ache, burning sensation in the head or other parts of the body, abdominal pain or discomfort. This phenomenon is also sometimes referred to as "Masked Depression" and is often seen in elderly patients coming to a physician clinic. Other features of depressed mood include, but are not limited to crying spells, sadness evidenced through facial expressions such as a constant frown and sometimes even by a lack of facial reactions to different stimuli.

The somatic or physical symptoms experienced by patients with depression are often referred to as neurovegetative symptoms. Several patients experience feeling unmotivated, feeling tired very often, find it difficult to complete assigned tasks or to engage in new work related or personal projects. Many patients report that they tend to wake up earlier than usual, and sometimes even several times during the night, leading to dissatisfaction with their sleep. Sleep complaints need to be addressed with the utmost priority, as most of the patients with depression usually report of some type of sleep disturbance and that these disturbances significantly contribute to their distress. Other neurovegetative symptoms also include menstrual irregularities in women and worsening of mood in the mornings.

The other hallmark feature of a depressive episode is Anhedonia. It is commonly described as a loss of interest. However, that is not an adequate description of the phenomenon. Therefore, the physician has to elicit that it is not merely a loss of interest, but in actuality is the loss of interest in a previously pleasurable activity. A good example would be that of a patient who enjoyed watching cricket matches live. His family members would even describe him as a die-hard cricket fan, but of recent he never seems to watch cricket matches, and once in a while only checks the scores online. When this patient is asked what happened by the doctor, he will often reply by saying that he just does not feel like watching live cricket anymore. This type of significant change in behavior is also significantly indicative of a morbid change in behavior likely to be due to a depressive illness.

Psychomotor changes are often observed in patients with depression. These could include *agitated behavior* in which a patient talks faster, appears restless, has frequent bodily behaviors such as hand wringing and hair pulling, and could also include the opposite type of behaviors such a slow reactions, *slowing of bodily movements*, increased response time or a drop in decision making ability (Psychomotor retardation).

Cognitive disturbances in depression include a poor evaluation of the patient himself, his future and the world around him. This is also often referred to as the *cognitive triad of depression*. These lead to faulty patterns in thinking further leading to problems such as *lowering of self-esteem* and confidence, feeling a lack of confidence in one's own time tested abilities, feeling helpless and hopeless, and in severe cases even wishing for death and thoughts to end one's life of this suffering (Suicidal Ideation).

The Greeks termed the word "*Melancholia*" a form of depression in which mood changes are accompanied by *measurable alterations in biological rhythms*. These biological factors include significant reductions in appetite, sleep and sexual functioning. These symptoms are even now clinically significant in several patients with depression. An equally prominent group of patients with depression often also experience the opposite such as increase in appetite, sleep as well as sexual functioning.

Anorexia and weight loss are often considered to be indicators of depression, but anorexia might be secondary to a decrease in the sensation of taste or more commonly a decrease in interest in eating food. It rarely could also be due to a morbid delusional belief that somebody has tampered with the food. Nutritional inadequacy could lead to severe unforeseen consequences and all medical practitioners must be weary of these symptoms. Any significant weight loss that occurs in the absence of any form of dieting or lifestyle modification must be investigated with the utmost priority.

Sexual dysfunction in depression often manifests as a decrease in desire to engage in any intimate sexual activity in both men and women. Depressed individuals do not respond adequately to sexual advances by the partner, and often vocally or otherwise also indicate that they do not wish to participate. Decreased libido in men can manifest as difficulty in achieving or maintaining an erection or sometimes even in spite of attaining erection men may not be satisfied with its quality. Females with depression sometimes experience a lack of internal lubrication or inability to achieve orgasm and sometimes in spite of reaching orgasm they are not satisfied with its quality and intensity. Men with depression often try to self-treat with advertised agents such as Sildenafil. Medical practitioners must exercise caution in these patients as many of the serotonergic drugs tend to aggravate sexual dysfunction with the exception of drugs like Bupropion and Buspirone. Sexual dysfunction should be addressed with the utmost seriousness, it can lead to significant interpersonal as well as marital conflicts.

A large portion of patients with depression also experience one or the other symptom of anxiety. Many patients report that they spend a lot of time worrying excessively about hypothetical future scenarios and this causes them a lot of distress. Patients also report feeling very restless and keep pacing around in their house. Many also experience several physical symptoms which cause them a lot of distress and make them repeatedly seek out medical help and evaluations. Some of these symptoms include:

- The feeling of heart pounding or racing
- Headaches, body aches, and abdominal discomfort
- Perspiration
- Feeling coldness in extremities
- Diarrhea
- Giddiness
- Nausea
- Goosebumps on the skin
- Feeling of choking or breathlessness
- Trembling of hands.

Patients often misinterpret these symptoms for a serious illness of the body and such patients often land up in the emergency room of the hospital requesting for a cardiac or respiratory evaluation. The thought of having a serious medical illness further contributes to distress and leads to worsening of mood. The high prevalence of symptoms of anxiety in patients with depression warrant adequate psychoeducation and addressal of the same.

A serious lack of understanding of mental illnesses accompanied by significant stigma about the same leads to several patients with depression going unrecognized and untreated. Due to a lack of understanding about the morbid changes happening in themselves because of the illness, patients often feel that they will never recover and lose all hopes of returning to their former selves. This often indicates a severe episode of depression.

Hopelessness leads to patients believing that ending their life is the only way out of their situation. Patients with suicidal intent may not express this desire directly. Some express it indirectly (I do not want to wake up from sleep), some patients are constantly tormented by a desire or urge to harm themselves. A small number of patients may even plan out the process carefully, including writing a note, preparing a will and taking out insurances. In some patients after starting initial treatment, once a psychomotor activity improves, but mood is still depressed, the risk of suicide may increase. This leads us to the conclusion that all persons with depression at any stage of treatment must be observed vigilantly by their family members or others.

A Delusion is defined as "A false, fixed and firm belief of morbid origin, that is out of keeping with a person's educational and cultural background, and is held with extraordinary conviction". In severe cases of depression, psychotic symptoms may present as delusions. The delusions are often related to a person's health, financial status, self-worth, and their interpersonal relationships. The delusions seen in these patients are those of guilt, worthlessness and often infidelity as well. A rare delusion in which a person feels as if he is dead inside or a walking corpse with rotting organs which is called Delusion of Nihilism is reported by some.

A severely depressed person may have a very low opinion of his or her own abilities leading to the feeling that his partner may leave them because of it. Psychotic features in depression also include the presence of hallucinations, which are false sensory perceptions, which occur in the absence of related stimulus in the environment, but their presence is again rare. These hallucinations are usually congruent to the mood of the patients and some patients report hearing accusatory voices about their mistakes causing further guilt and distress to the patient.

Another important aspect every clinician needs to understand is that depression does not clinically present in the same manner in children, adolescents, adult and in older people. Most of the features described in this chapter are likely to be seen in adult patients, but children often will display a different clinical picture. In children and adolescents, academic decline will very commonly be present. There can also be displays of excessive clinging behavior to parents or caregivers, social withdrawal, refusal in participating in the play, refusing to go to school or do homework can be some of the different presentations of depression in children. Adolescent depression can present truancy, substance use or engaging in antisocial behavior.

When older persons are concerned, it is worthwhile to note that they are more vulnerable to suffering from a depressive episode. Presence of medical morbidity, poor social support, neglect, substance use and financial stressors and treatment with certain drugs increase the likelihood of developing a depressive episode. Depression in the elderly may manifest as chronic dissatisfaction with life. Prominent symptoms commonly observed are those of reduced energy, appetite loss, excessive pre-occupation with bodily symptoms or general health and low self-esteem. Some patients may also present with suicidal ideation or paranoid ideation. The presence of a dementing disorder or other psychiatric morbidity causes further difficult in demarcating the symptoms of depression. Therefore, geriatric patients need to be given special attention and should be evaluated thoroughly.

SUGGESTED READING

1. Akiskal HS. Mood disorders. In: Sadock BJ, Sadock VA, Ruiz P (Eds). Kaplan & Sadock's Comprehensive Textbook of Psychiatry. 10th edition. Philadelphia, Pennsylvania, USA: Wolters Kluwer; 2017.
2. Kalin NH. The critical relationship between anxiety and depression. Am J Psychiatry. 2020;177(5):365-7.
3. Murrough JW, Iacoviello B, Neumeister A, Charney DS, Iosifescu DV. Cognitive dysfunction in depression: neurocircuitry and new therapeutic strategies. Neurobiol Learn Mem. 2011;96(4):553-63.
4. Perlis RH, Brown E, Baker RW, Nierenberg AA. Clinical features of bipolar depression versus major depressive disorder in large multicenter trials. Am J Psychiatry. 2006;163(2):225-31.

CHAPTER 4: Diagnosis of Depression

Nikhil Gurjar

INTRODUCTION

Depression presents in a lot of different ways clinically. Classically the descriptions of depression have been that of a person with a downward gaze, appearing sad with sluggish movements, but as discussed in the previous chapter that is not always the case. Sadness is a normal reaction to many situations in life and can be misunderstood to be a depressive illness. Additionally, the clinical picture of depression may vary depending on the severity and chronicity of the illness. Therefore, it is essential to understand how to correctly diagnose depression in a standardized acceptable manner.

Depression with its vast and complex presentations can often be tricky to correctly diagnose and can further lead to worsening of a patient's quality of life. It is also important to understand the diagnostic criteria to prevent mistaking a normal emotional reaction from a pathological mood state. Several diagnostic criteria for the same have been proposed and the popularly used ones include those given by the American Psychiatric Association and the World Health Organization.

CORE FEATURES

To make a diagnosis of depression the core features of depression, i.e., depressed or low mood for a significant portion of the day, anhedonia (loss of interest in previously pleasurable activities) and easy fatiguability must be present. As these are the core symptoms of depression, at least 1 or 2 of these must be present for a minimum period of 2 weeks.

FREQUENTLY CO-OCCURRING SYMPTOMS

Besides the core symptoms of the illness, there are other frequently co-occurring symptoms that are present in many patients. These include changes in appetite, weight loss (more than a 5% change in body weight), sleep disturbances in the form of insomnia or excessive sleep, psychomotor agitation or slowing.

COGNITIVE SYMPTOMS

Cognitive symptoms such as a decrease in attention span, difficulty in concentration and indecisiveness are also commonly present. Feelings of worthlessness, excessive guilt or self-blame, recurrent thoughts of death or plans to end one's own life are some of the thought related symptoms that may be present.

GENERAL CONSIDERATIONS WHILE MAKING A DIAGNOSIS

Besides the core features of depression, at least 3 or 4 more from the other symptoms must be present to make a diagnosis of depression. Additionally, the presence of symptoms must also cause a decline in the level of a person's social and occupational functioning. The symptoms should not be secondary to any organic brain illness, a general medical condition or any substance or drug. Presence of other major psychiatric morbidities such as bipolar disorder, schizophrenia or delusional disorder must be ruled out before proceeding to make a diagnosis of depression.

FEATURES OF A MIXED MOOD STATE

Besides the general features of depression, features of anxiety such as feeling excessively tense, very often, feeling restless and unable to sit at one place, or excessive worrying may be present. Sometimes depression may also present with mixed mood features which include a pervasive irritable or expansile mood, grandiose thoughts or behavior, rapid pressurized speech and over religiosity and overspending. Sometimes melancholic features such as a lack of reactivity to pleasurable stimulus, early morning awakenings, severe anhedonia may also be present.

OTHER ATYPICAL FEATURES

Depression may also present with atypical features such as overeating, oversleeping and feeling of heaviness in the body.

These abovementioned symptoms are not required to make a diagnosis of depression, but they must be noted clinically as they help in better management of the patient. The core and general symptoms of depression are of key consideration while making a diagnosis. The onset of these symptoms is at times acute, but may often also be insidious. Clinically it sometimes becomes a challenge to demarcate the exact onset of symptoms. Additional importance must be given to elicit suicidal thoughts or plans or death wishes as they often indicate higher severity of depression, and these patients require intensive patient care and management. Any other general medical comorbidity must also be addressed as worsening of one may result in worsening of the other.

Once a clinical diagnosis is made which satisfies the diagnostic criteria, the symptom severity must also be assessed. It is very important to understand the symptom severity of patient as it helps us decide if the patient can be treated on a outpatient basis or if he/she may require to be treated on a inpatient basis at a psychiatric center. If a person has mild to moderate symptoms, he/she may be treated on a outpatient basis. Severe patients or those presenting with suicidal thoughts or behavior require intensive inpatient treatment. Even patients with moderate symptoms with a high degree of social and occupational impairment may benefit from inpatient services.

To assess symptom severity, several different psychometric assessment scales are used. These scales are usually in the form of questionnaires which assess symptoms of the disorder on which they are based, some of the popular tools used for assessing depression are:

- Hamilton Depression Rating Scale
- Montgomery-Asberg Depression Rating Scale
- Becks Depression Inventory
- Zung Self-Rating Depression Scale.

Psychometric scales are both clinician rated and patient rated (self-rated). It is always advisable to use a combination of both. Doing so can help in under-standing the patient better in a objective as well as subjective manner. Using only clinician rated tools may sometimes not give an adequate idea of the patients suffering, and using only patient rated instruments can cause under/over estimation of the severity of symptoms.

Additionally, there are several tools available to assess suicidality specifically in patients. This helps us in understanding the risk of further attempts better and results in better patient care and reduced mortality or harm to the patient. Some of these tools include:

- Columbia Suicide Severity Rating Scale
- Beck Scale for Suicidal Ideation.

Psychiatric rating scales should be used from time to time during the course of treatment. It helps us understand the improvement shown by the patient better. Even patients upon seeing the improvement in the scores of the test feel a sense of satisfaction which will further contribute to improving the doctor patient relationship and will also help in building trust in the plan of management. Ideally the rating scales must be used till the patient is in recovery and may be used for the last time when clinician wants to take a decision on tapering or stopping medications.

SUGGESTED READING

1. Fremouw WJ, De Perczel M, Ellis TE. Suicide risk: Assessment and response guidelines. Pergamon Press; 1990.
2. Smith KM, Renshaw PF, Bilello J. The diagnosis of depression: current and emerging methods. Compr Psychiatry. 2013;54(1):1-6.

Approach to Management of a Patient with Depression

Jatin Anand

■ INTRODUCTION

Depression is a common psychiatric disorder contributing to the global burden of disease. It is associated with poor quality of life and impairment in socio-occupational functioning. According to previous studies by the WHO, depression was the fourth leading cause of disability. However, after the COVID-19 pandemic, depression is thought to be one of the topmost leading causes of disability. It has increased the cost of healthcare and is associated with longer duration of hospitalization, poor cooperation and compliance with treatment and high rates of morbidity. Due to the stigma attached with psychiatric illnesses, patients often hesitate to visit a psychiatrist. In the larger interest of patients, it is important for general physicians to be well versed with the treatment protocols laid down for depression so that management can be initiated early.

■ EVALUATION AND ASSESSMENT

A comprehensive assessment of depression is required before initiating management of depression. This includes a detailed history from both patient and family, physical examination, and mental state examinations.

There are three core features of depression which include symptoms suggestive of low mood, loss of interest or pleasure in activities that are normally enjoyable and having low energy or feeling fatigued. Other features include decreased concentration, low self-esteem and confidence, ideas of guilt and feeling unworthy, bleak, pessimistic views of the future, ideas or acts of self-harm or suicide, decreased or disturbed sleep and decreased appetite. For a patient to be diagnosed with depression, one must make sure that these symptoms have been persistent for at least 2 weeks and are causing psychosocial dysfunction.

It is not necessary that a patient will present only with the symptoms mentioned above. There can be instances where the patient might initially present with complaints of generalized body ache and fatigue, but on evaluation underlying features of depression can be revealed. At times, certain atypical features such as increased sleep and appetite may be present. In severe cases, a patient can present with anxiety or even psychotic symptoms such as the presence of delusions and hallucinations.

It is important to note that whenever a diagnosis of depression is suspected, always rule out bipolar disorder by detailed history taking of the patient and the family because the antidepressants used in management can induce a switch to manic phase. Some signs which can indicate the presence of a bipolar disorder include the presence of psychotic features, atypical signs such as increased sleep and appetite, irritability, early age of onset and a positive family history of bipolar disorders.

Treatment history, if any, should be evaluated thoroughly for the kind of medication used along with the dosage, compliance, response to treatment and any adverse effects reported.

A thorough evaluation of depression can be supplemented with ratings on standardized scales of assessment such as Hamilton's or Beck's Depression Inventory.

During evaluation, it is important to obtain a history of substance abuse/dependence and medical illnesses which are commonly associated with depression. Certain medications are known to cause depression.

INVESTIGATIONS

Routine investigations can be carried out to rule out other medical illnesses. Neuroimaging is indicated in elderly patients having their first episode and in patients exhibiting neurological signs.

TREATMENT SETTING

Usually, most patients can be managed on OPD basis, but some patients do require in-patient care. Some of these indications are presently of suicidal behavior, refusal to eat or malnutrition. It is essential that family caregivers are present during inpatient admission.

The key to successful treatment of major depressive disorder lies in ensuring compliance with treatment. Issues such as apprehension regarding adverse effects, poor motivation and lackadaisical attitude should be resolved to prevent non-adherence and subsequent relapse.

INITIAL TREATMENT

For mild to moderate cases of depression, either pharmacotherapy or psychotherapy or a combination of both can be used. Severe cases usually require exclusive pharmacotherapy. Some of the most common psychotherapies being used currently have been listed in **Table 1** below.

TABLE 1: Common psychotherapy modalities	
Cognitive behavior therapy	Identifying problems, cognitive distortions/errors, generating alternative thoughts, replacing unwanted behaviors with productive behaviors, anxiety management strategies, and relaxation techniques
Interpersonal therapy	Focuses on losses, problems with roles in relationships, and analysis of social skills deficits leading to interpersonal friction
Supportive psychotherapy	Allowing patient to ventilate, facilitation of providing a safe environment, providing emotional support, guidance increasing patient's self-esteem, and increasing hope
Behavior therapy	Training in social skills, roleplay, scheduling activities and designing schedules for the day, help in problem solving
Marital therapy	Behavioral exchange, improving spousal communication by encouraging open non-judgmental talk about issues, and resolution of conflict around common issues
Family therapy	The principles used are similar to marital therapy, however they usually involve all of the immediate and close family members

Pharmacotherapy

The choice of medication depends upon patient preference, previous history of response to a particular drug, past adverse effects, cost, history of other medication, age and comorbidities.

Some commonly used antidepressants along with their recommended dosages are listed in **Table 2**.

TABLE 2: Commonly prescribed antidepressants		
Antidepressant	Usual dose range (mg/day)	Common side effects
Selective serotonin reuptake inhibitors (SSRIs)		
Escitalopram	10–20	Sexual dysfunction such as delayed ejaculation, loss of libido, erectile dysfunction, gastrointestinal (GI) dysfunction such as constipation, belching, indigestion, weight gain, anxiety, and insomnia
Sertraline	50–200	
Fluoxetine	20–80	
Fluvoxamine	50–300	
Paroxetine	20–60	
Serotonin norepinephrine reuptake inhibitors (SNRIs)		
Venlafaxine	75–300	Mild anticholinergic effects such as dry mouth, blurring of vision, drowsiness, GI distress, and headache
Desvenlafaxine	50–100	
Duloxetine	20–60	

Contd...

Contd...

Antide-pressant	Usual dose range (mg/day)	Common side effects
Noradrenaline and specific serotonin antidepressants (NaSSAs)		
Mirtazapine	7.5–45	Mild anticholinergic effects, sedation, lethargy, flatulence, indigestion, weight gain, and orthostasis
Tricyclic antidepressants (TCAs)		
Amitriptyline	50–200	Sexual dysfunction, anticholinergic side effects, drowsiness, orthostasis, mild GI distress, and weight gain
Nortriptyline	25–150	
Clomipramine	50–300	
Imipramine	50–300	
Desipramine	75–300	
Doxepin	50–300	
Atypical antidepressants		
Trazodone	100–300	Mild anticholinergic side effects, drowsiness, orthostasis, mild GI distress, weight gain, severe hepatotoxicity, priapism
Nefazodone	100–300	

Contd...

Contd...

Antide-pressant		Usual dose range (mg/day)	Common side effects
Unicyclic antidepressants			
	Bupropion	150–450	Mild GI distress, possible worsening of psychotic symptoms, sleep disturbances, high-risk of seizures beyond 450 mg/day
Serotonin partial agonist reuptake inhibitor (SPARI)			
	Vilazodone	20–40	Nausea/vomiting, diarrhea, insomnia

After deciding on an antidepressant, start the drug at lower dosage to minimize the initial adverse effect and gradually increase it till the desired effect is achieved. During the initial phase of treatment, antidepressants may be supplemented with benzodiazepines or other hypnotics to allay associated symptoms of anxiety and insomnia. Ensure proper compliance with medication before assessing treatment response after 4-6 weeks.

An improvement of more than 50% requires continuing treatment at the same dosage. If the patient reports a 25-50% improvement during the first 4-6 weeks, optimize the dosage of the antidepressant to the maximum tolerable dose.

Whenever using higher doses, closely monitor the patients, an increase in severity of adverse effects or the emergence of newer side effects.

If no improvement (<25%) is reported, consider changing the medication. A thorough review and reappraisal of diagnosis may also be considered. Most commonly, a different antidepressant, is used in patients who have not responded to the prescribed treatment. The newer medication can be of the same pharmacologic class (e.g., from one SSRI to another SSRI) or to a drug from a different pharmacologic class (e.g., from one SSRI to tricyclic antidepressant).

Augmentation

Alternatively, medication may be augmented with other agents, which includes adding a second antidepressant from a different pharmacologic class or adding an adjunctive drug such as lithium, anticonvulsants etc.

Patients having suboptimal responses can also be supplemented with psychotherapy (cognitive behavior therapy, interpersonal therapy, supportive psychotherapy), yoga and meditation. Electroconvulsive therapy can be considered in severe depression with suicidal thoughts or where pharmacological measures are ineffective.

Measures to improve medication compliance:
- Teach patient when and how often to take medicines
- Preferably give once a day dosing
- Prescribe minimum number of tablets
- Ask patients for formulation preference (tablet, capsule etc.)
- Explain the patient that beneficial effects will be seen after 2-4 weeks of medication
- Explain the patient the need to take medication even after feeling better.

- Explanation of side effects, reporting side effects and what to do
- Consult doctor before discontinuing medication.

Treatment Resistant Depression

Around 20-30% of patients fail to achieve a satisfactory response. In some cases, it can be due to faulty diagnosis, noncompliance or additional factors such as coexisting psychiatric and general medical conditions. Always reassess the diagnosis and treatment in terms of dosage, duration and compliance before proceeding further. Some clinicians have advocated two successive trials of medications of different pharmacologic categories for adequate duration before diagnosing treatment resistant depression (TRD). Management of TRD includes adding adjunctive medication like lithium and T3 hormone, combining two antidepressants and using somatic treatments such as electroconvulsive therapy (ECT) and Repetitive transcranial magnetic stimulation (rTMS).

ADVERSE EFFECTS

To ensure compliance with the medication, it is important to educate the patient regarding common unwanted side effects of frequently used antidepressants. These include gastrointestinal side effects such as nausea, GI disturbances such as diarrhea and constipation, flatulence, indigestion, autonomic side effects such as excessive night sweats and dry mouth, sexual adverse effects such as decreased libido, delayed ejaculation, and sleep disturbances such as insomnia or feeling drowsy. Other adverse effects include bleeding tendencies, hyponatremia, weight gain, risk of diabetes and QTc prolongation. Many of the above adverse effects are self-limiting in nature. If they persist, symptomatic treatment can be initiated to mitigate these effects.

CONTINUATION AND MAINTENANCE OF TREATMENT

The aim is to maintain the gains achieved in the acute phase of treatment and prevent relapse of symptoms. Studies have shown that 50–85% of patients with a single episode of major depression go on to experience at least another episode in their lifetime. Hence, it has been suggested that treatment initiated in the acute phase should be continued at the same dose for at least 16–24 weeks. Supportive psychotherapy and other modalities such as ECT and yoga can also be used during this phase. The duration between follow-ups can be reduced gradually as dictated by response to treatment.

The total duration of treatment depends upon the past history of depressive episodes and previous treatment history. In all, several studies have demonstrated that a total effective treatment period lasts anywhere from 6–9 months in order to prevent relapses. However, there is no consensus regarding the duration of treatment. Patients with a history of three or more relapses require long-term treatment.

DISCONTINUATION OF TREATMENT

Patients often desire to discontinue medication after a prolonged period of treatment, which is attributable to myths surrounding psychiatric medications causing dependence. It is important for physicians to remove such misconceptions. Treatment can be discontinued taking into consideration the probability of recurrence, frequency and severity of past depressive episodes, persistence of symptoms even after recovery, comorbid chronic medical illnesses and patient preference. Rather than discontinuing the medications abruptly, it is advisable to taper the medications over several weeks to months in order to minimize discontinuation symptoms. These include flu-like symptoms, disturbed sleep, nausea and agitation. Such symptoms are more common with medications having shorter half-lives such as paroxetine, venlafaxine and TCAs. These medications require longer, more gradual tapering.

Mild symptoms require simple reassurance as these are self-limiting. If symptoms are not relieved, symptomatic treatment with analgesics, antiemetics and anxiolytics can be started. Severe symptoms require restarting antidepressants and tapering the dose even more slowly.

Patients should be taught how to identify early signs of depression, so that future relapses can be controlled with early intervention. It is better to monitor patients for a few months after discontinuing treatment in order to identify relapse.

ANTIDEPRESSANT INDUCED SWITCH TO MANIC STATE

Persons with underlying bipolar disorder may experience a switch to a manic state upon administration of an antidepressant drug. The warning signs for this switch include a rapid response in depressive symptoms, increase in rate of speech, overactivity, grandiose thinking, increase in risk taking behavior, increased goal directed activity, overfamiliarity, disinhibited behavior, impulsive behavior and physical aggression which may be unprovoked. In this case, medical practitioners must take note that it is very likely that person is suffering from bipolar disorder, and should immediately stop the antidepressant agent. If a person presents with agitation and/or assaultive behavior, he must immediately be referred to an inpatient psychiatric care facility as he or she may pose a threat to themselves or others.

SUGGESTED READING

1. Gelenberg AJ, Freeman MP, Markowitz JC, Rosenbaum JF, Thase ME, Trivedi MH, et al. American Psychiatric Association practice guidelines for the treatment of patients with major depressive disorder. Am J Psychiatry. 2010;167(Suppl 10):9-118.
2. Kupfer DJ. The pharmacological management of depression. Dialogues Clin Neurosci. 2005;7(3):191-205.
3. National Collaborating Centre for Mental Health (UK. Depression: The Treatment and Management of Depression in Adults (Updated Edition). British Psychological Society; 2010. PMID:22132433.
4. Timonen M, Liukkonen T. Management of depression in adults. BMJ. 2008;336(7641):435-9.

CHAPTER 6

Suicidality in Context of Depression: The Do's and Don'ts

Jatin Anand

■ SUICIDE

Suicide is one of the leading causes of death in India. According to latest studies, more than 1.5 lakh suicides were reported in India during 2020, which roughly translates to 17 people dying every hour. The overall male to female ratio of suicide victims is roughly 70:30. Most common age groups impacted are 18–30 years of age and 30–45 years of age. The most common means of suicide have been hanging, poisoning and drowning.

General practitioners are frequently in charge of treating patients who have suicide attempts, since not every hospital is equipped with psychiatric emergency services. Hence, it is essential that general practitioners have a well-defined plan in place for such patients encountered in either the clinic, hospital or the emergency department to provide immediate care, support and guidance.

Once this is done, it will be possible to evaluate the attempt's history, conditions, and likelihood of repetition.

In this chapter, the evaluation criteria for suicide risk have been reviewed, with a clear focus on establishing a doctor-patient relationship to improve the patient's condition and to prevent future suicide attempts.

DIFFERENTIATING FROM PARASUICIDE

Parasuicide refers to the act of self-harm without the realistic expectation of death. These are also commonly known as suicidal gestures. The main difference between "true attempt" and parasuicide is that in the former, there is clear intent with the expectation of death. However, such gestures can occasionally be fatal due to miscalculations or unexpected outcomes of the attempt. In the emergency setting, it can be challenging to gauge the patient's intent. Hence, it is advisable to give the benefit of doubt to such patients and leave no stone unturned in the care of such patients.

INITIAL MANAGEMENT

The patient may present to the general practitioner with either overt complaints of having suicidal thoughts or patient might come with other complaints and during the course of the interview, the practitioner may find them to be harboring suicidal thoughts. In both the situations, it is important for the physician to fully assess the patient regarding the intent behind the suicidal thoughts, any medical or psychiatric history and the immediate family support. The patient may be referred to a psychiatrist for further management, but quite often, due to lack of emergency psychiatric services, the physician has to take on this role and manage such patients initially.

Any patient who has attempted suicide should be first stabilized medically using protocols devised for such emergency based on Advanced Cardiac Life Support and vital sign stabilization.

Patients posing a risk to themselves, or others can be restrained either physically or chemically. Strict antisuicidal measures such as removal of sharp objects, medicines, medical equipment and other potentially harmful objects should be removed from the immediate vicinity and the patient should be isolated.

Such patients whenever admitted should be allocated a bed which is visible from the nursing station. Preferably, an attendant should be present with such patients on a regular basis.

■ INTERVIEW

Once the patient has stabilized, the next step is to establish a history. The environment for such interviews should be comfortable for the patient. Preferably, interview the patient alone at first as they might be hesitant in front of their family and friends. It is important for the practitioner to remain calm and non-judgmental during the interview. The practitioner should express empathy toward the patient and engage with the patient actively. The interview can start with a simple question such as "How may I help you today?". Always pay attention to the patients' replies for evaluating the precipitating factors behind the attempt. In case of patients not opening up about their attempt, focus on the reasons behind their reluctance. A simple question such as "Why now?" can help shed some of the hesitance. Try to establish the important people in the patient's life by asking questions like who will they leave behind. Evaluate the emotional state and reiterate their issues. For patients expressing hopelessness, death seems to be a quick fix for all their issues and helps them avoid pain and stress in their lives. Empathy helps the patient to trust the practitioner and helps initiate a belief that circumstances can get better. The aim is for the patient to believe that the physician understands their situation and distress.

The interview should also explore the past history of any medication or substance use and the support system to which the patient will be returning to. The physician should obtain a detailed medical history, including any chronic comorbid medical illness and family history for medical and psychiatric illness.

ASSESSMENT OF DEGREE OF SUICIDALITY

Suicidal ideation is an important determinant of risk as it precedes suicide. The majority of patients with suicidal ideation will not die by suicide, hence the physician should evaluate all factors that may increase the risk for suicide. The physician should determine the presence, magnitude and persistence of current and past suicidal ideation. It is important to understand that the absence of suicidal ideation does not remove the risk for suicidal behavior, since some individuals will outrightly deny such ideas when asked directly. A common myth which needs to be addressed is that asking about suicidal ideation increases the risk of suicide.

Patients who have a strong suicidal ideation often develop a suicide plan, the formulation of which typically happens within one year of developing such ideas. A typical suicide plan includes the method of harm, timing, availability of method, procuring required items and a rehearsal. The more detailed and specific the plan, the greater is the suicide risk. High risk behavior includes using lethal methods and going out of the way to avoid detection.

Two domains which need to be assessed are lethality and intentionality. Lethality refers to the likelihood that death will occur if one of the methods to die by suicide is used. Some examples of methods suggestive of high lethality include hanging, jumping, self-immolation. Low lethality methods include wrist cutting and overdosing on non-prescription drugs such as paracetamol. Suicidal intent refers to the patient's subjective expectations and desire to die due to self-inflicted injury. These expectations may or may not correspond to the lethality of an attempt. The subjective belief about the lethality of a method is more important than the objective lethality of the chosen method.

The presence of a suicide note also indicates premeditation and greater suicidal intent. The physician should assess the content and timing of any suicide note retrieved and should include it in the medical record. Collateral information from the paramedical staff, friends and family is also important regarding the timing and sequence of events. This can aid in deciding methods of treatment.

MENTAL STATUS AND PHYSICAL EXAMINATION

A physician should be observant during the entire interview regarding any abnormality regarding mental status. Simple observations like whether the patient is aware about the day of the week, identifying the place and the people around him can shed light on the patient's level of alertness and orientation. Rule out mood and psychotic symptoms such as delusions. These preliminary findings can help the psychiatrist in formulating a management plan later on.

As a physician, conduct a thorough physical examination with special emphasis on physical findings associated with chronic disease, alcoholism and other substance abuse. Observe the general appearance and behavior, dressing, grooming and level of hygiene. Examine the body for needle marks, excoriations and unusual odors, which can be indicative of past abuse or injury.

Proper documentation of the interview, including the assessment, differential diagnosis and treatment plan is a must. If possible, a psychiatric consultation is preferred.

DISCHARGE

Before discharging the patient, do arrange for a psychiatric consultation to rule out psychiatric illnesses which might have been missed during the initial evaluation. It is important to educate the close contacts or attendants regarding anti-suicidal measures previously mentioned and ensure a regular follow-up with the treating physician. The risk of another suicide attempt is highest during the time of discharge.

CONTINUED TREATMENT AND FOLLOW-UPS

A close working relationship between the patient and the treating physician will ensure appropriate recovery and decrease the chance of future suicide attempts. This relationship depends on the physician's knowledge of the patient's physical and psychosocial circumstances. Depressed patients have higher incidence rates of chronic medical illnesses, hence they visit their primary physician frequently. The physician can monitor such high-risk patients on a regular basis.

Hence, it is important to identify vulnerable patients based on identifying high- risk factors as mentioned below.

High-risk factors in assessing suicide risk:
- Past suicide attempts
- Seriousness of previous attempts
- Family history of suicide
- Feelings of hopelessness
- Substance abuse
- Social isolation
- Personal or family history of psychiatric illness
- History of loss
- Preoccupation with death.

Some clinicians have also suggested "no-suicide" contracts in managing suicidal patients, asking them to commit verbally or in writing to not act on suicidal impulses, but instead contact a source of help such as the primary care physician or suicide helplines. The patient feels that their physician is concerned regarding their health and also gives them a concrete plan to follow during a crisis. It does not fully ensure patient safety, but if the patient does not agree to this contract, consider hospitalization.

Close follow up is a must and psychiatric referral should be done at the earliest. The physician should help remove the stigma and misconceptions surrounding mental illnesses, so that patients can seek psychiatric help.

Medication can play a significant role in the management of patients who are having suicidal ideation or have attempted suicide. Medication usually includes antidepressants such as selective serotonin reuptake inhibitors like escitalopram and sertraline.

An important point to keep in mind is that antidepressant medicines can "activate" depressed individuals, which in turn increases the risk of suicidal behavior. Activation means that patient may experience a transient increase in anxiety, restlessness, agitation and sleep disturbances. This needs to be addressed by psycho-educating the patient about these symptoms, and to prevent them a cover of benzodiazepines for low doses for a few days can be given. Hence, patients who have been initiated on medication need to be closely monitored.

SUGGESTED READING

1. D'Anci KE, Uhl S, Giradi G, Martin C. Treatments for the prevention and management of suicide: a systematic review. Ann Intern Med. 2019;171(5):334-42.
2. Mann JJ, Apter A, Bertolote J, Beautrais A, Currier D, Haas A, et al. Suicide prevention strategies: a systematic review. Jama. 2005;294(16):2064-74.
3. Panesar B, Soni D, Khan MI, Bdair F, Holek M, Tahir T, et al. National suicide management guidelines recommending family-based prevention, intervention and postvention and their association with suicide mortality rates: systematic review. BJ Psych Open. 2022;8(2):e54.
4. Simon RI, Hales RE. The American Psychiatric Publishing Textbook of Suicide Assessment and Management. American Psychiatric Pub; 2012.

Index

A

Abdominal discomfort 17
Advanced cardiac
life support 39
American Psychiatric
Association 21
Amitriptyline 31
Anhedonia 3, 22
Anorexia 16
Anticholinergic side effects 31
Antidepressants 30-32, 36
   assessment of degree of 31
Anxiety 30
   symptom of 17
Atrophy 7
Augmentation 33

B

Beck scale for suicidal
ideation 25
Becks depression inventory 24
Behavior therapy 29
Belching 30
Biogenic amines 6
Body aches 17
Breathlessness 17
Bupropion 32

C

Cerebrospinal fluid 6
Choking, feeling of 17
Clomipramine 31
Cognitive behavior therapy 29
Columbia suicide severity
rating scale 25
Constipation 30
COVID-19 pandemic 26

D

Delusion 18
Depressed mood 13
Depression 1, 2, 10, 12, 16,
19-21, 23, 26, 27, 34
   clinical features of 12
   cognitive theory of 9
   comprehensive assessment
of 26
   context of 38
   diagnosis of 21
   etiology of 5
   salient features of 3
Depressive disorder 3, 8
Desipramine 31
Desvenlafaxine 30
Diarrhea 17, 32
Doxepin 31
Drowsiness 30, 31
Dry mouth 30
Duloxetine 30

E

Ejaculation, delayed 30
Electroconvulsive therapy
33, 34
Energy, lack of 3
Erectile dysfunction 30
Escitalopram 30

F

Feeling coldness 17
Flatulence 31
Fluoxetine 30
Fluvoxamine 30

G

Gastrointestinal distress 30
   mild 31, 32
Gastrointestinal dysfunction 30
Giddiness 17

H

Hamilton depression rating scale 24
Hamilton's or Beck's depression inventory 28
Hands, trembling of 17
Headache 17, 30
Heart, feeling of 17
Hepatotoxicity, severe 31
Hopelessness, feeling of 44
Hypercortisolism 8
Hypothalamic pituitary adrenal axis 7

I

Imipramine 31
Immune dysfunction 8
Indigestion 30, 31
Insomnia 30, 32
Interpersonal therapy 29

L

Lethargy 31
Libido, loss of 30

M

Major depressive disorder 12
Marital therapy 29
Masked depression 14
Melancholia 15
Mental status 42
Mild anticholinergic effects 30, 31
Mirtazapine 31
Montgomery-Asberg depression rating scale 24
Mood
   disorders 5
   sadness of 3

N

Nausea 17, 32
Nefazodone 31
Nihilism, delusion of 19
Nortriptyline 31

O

Orthostasis 31

P

Parasuicide 39
Parkinson disease 6
Paroxetine 30
Pharmacotherapy 30
Pleasure, loss of 3
Priapism 31
Psychometric scales 24
Psychomotor retardation 15

R

Repetitive transcranial magnetic stimulation 34
Reserpine 6

S

Sedation 31
Seizures, high-risk of 32
Selective serotonin reuptake inhibitors 30
Serotonin
    metabolites 6
    norepinephrine reuptake inhibitors 30, 32
Sertraline 30
Sexual dysfunction 16, 31
Sildenafil 17
Sleep
    disturbances 32
    lack of 3
Substance abuse 44
Suicidal gestures 39
Suicidal ideation 15
Suicidality 38
    assessment of degree of 41
Suicide 38
    family history of 44
Supportive psychotherapy 29

T

Thyroid-stimulating hormone 7

Trazodone 31
Tricyclic antidepressant 31, 33

U

Unicyclic antidepressants 32

V

Venlafaxine 30
Vilazodone 32
Vision, blurring of 30
Vital sign stabilization 39
Vomiting 32

W

Weight
    gain 30, 31
    loss 16
World Health Organization 1, 21

Z

Zung self-rating depression scale 24